T0381208

# From My Garden to My Kitchen

*Favorite Creations and Recreations*

Angelia Ross-Little

*AuthorHouse™*
*1663 Liberty Drive*
*Bloomington, IN 47403*
*www.authorhouse.com*
*Phone: 1 (800) 839-8640*

*Published by AuthorHouse 08/03/2015*

*ISBN: 978-1-5049-1561-8 (sc)*
*ISBN: 978-1-5049-1562-5 (e)*

*Library of Congress Control Number: 2015909976*

*Print information available on the last page.*

*Any people depicted in stock imagery provided by Thinkstock are models, and such images are being used for illustrative purposes only. Certain stock imagery © Thinkstock.*

*This book is printed on acid-free paper.*

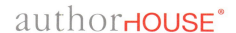

# ACKNOWLEDGEMENTS

I want to thank my Mother who is the light in my life. She has always supported me in all my ventures and goals and gives me her feedback and so often, her help in the kitchen.

My cousin Nina who actually put the cookbook idea in my head, she is also one of my biggest fans and that means a lot to me! My friends and Co-workers who have often been my testers without ever questioning what they were about to eat, they don't even ask any more, they eat it and then I tell. You know who you are and it means a lot to me!

*I Dedicate This First Cookbook to my Dad!*

So, finally I decided to sit down and do this. I love to cook and have for as long as I can remember. I have always been interested in cooking and creating recipes. At 12 or 13 years old watching Julia Child, Graham Kerr aka "The Galloping Gourmet," and other chefs on television instead of the usually popular shows during that time, I am certain part of my future had already been determined.

Back in the day, I hung out with a very awesome crew. We would have a party to celebrate every holiday that was a day off from work. President's Day, Martin Luther King's birthday, 4th of July, Labor Day, Columbus Day, and Veteran's Day were usually three-day weekends when I lived in Boston and we would always plan a get-together. I did most of the cooking. Happily I might add. A typical menu might be Stir Fried Rice with Vegetables aka Dirty Rice, Quiche Lorraine, Honey-Baked Chicken Wings with Tarragon, Sautéed Pork with Apples and an assortment of "starters" i.e. Mushrooms stuffed with Crabmeat. I discovered the wonderful combination of cream cheese and crabmeat in baking as well. For our annual Christmas Breakfast, my specialty was always baked eggs with sautéed vegetables and homemade apple sauce. My mom would fry some porgies; cook some grits, ham, bacon sausage, hash browns.

Our Annual Christmas Breakfast was a tradition started with by my Aunt Mae, and passed on to my Mother. What began with an invitation to a few family members and friends in 1975, ended with 45 people attending our last Christmas Breakfast in 2003.

After moving to the South 10 years ago, I've rediscovered my joy of cooking and want to share this joy with those who "LOVE TO COOK!" I am not a chef…I JUST LOVE TO COOK!

You will not find calorie counts or nutritional information in this cookbook because all of my recipes are nutritional and everything should be eaten in moderation, always drink a lot of water and exercise as much and as often as you can.

Feel free to do your own thing; if you choose to use 1 tablespoon of unsalted butter and my recipe calls for 2 – go for it. I use lots of herbs, of which mostly come from my own herb garden, garlic and real butter (unsalted of course), and always fresh ingredients.

Well, here is it…. Hope you enjoy using and reading this cookbook as much as I enjoyed writing it.

# Table of Contents

# Before You Start

1.  Always read the recipe all the way through to be sure you have all the necessary ingredients.

2.  Check your recipe the day before incase preparations need to be made the day before, like marinating.

3.  Chop all the vegetables and herbs you will be using in your recipe and set them aside. Such as, onions, garlic, etc.

4.  Gather all your ingredients and place aside – this goes for any utensils, pots & pans you will need.

5.  Preheat your oven if you need to bake.

6.  If you are without a dishwasher, I find it helpful to wash your dishes as you finish with them. This leaves less clean up when you are done

7.  I find it helpful to write out my menu, the cooking times, and in what order I am going to prepare my dishes.

# A Few of my Cooking Tips

**GARLIC** – when chopping or mincing garlic, wet knife and fingers to keep the garlic from sticking to your knife or fingers.

**CUTTING BOARDS** – Have separate cutting boards, one for meats, another for vegetables, fruit and herbs and another if you chop a lot of hot pepper. Always wash your boards and dry them thoroughly before storing, especially the one you use for meat.

**SPICES**: Store your spices in a cool, dry place; heat and humidity cause herbs and spices to lose their flavors. I keep my expensive items like Saffron and Cardamom on a shelf in the refrigerator.

**THE BEST**: When possible use the best quality herbs, spices, olive oils, extract and vinegars. Balsamic vinegar should be aged at least 5 years; I generally will not purchase one less than 8 years. A good Balsamic can be costly, but if you use it for salads, it is worth it.

**BRINING**: Brine your poultry and pork; this will assure that your cooked product will be moist, tender and full of flavor.

**PREPARATION**: Cut, chopped & mince all the items you will need for your recipe. Place them in little containers and set them aside so they are ready when you are. Have the spices you will need handy; avoid trips back and forth to the cabinet.

**BAKING**: Eggs should always be at room temperature.

**MEAT**: When cooking steak, let your meat come to room temperature before placing it on heat. This will avoid the meat being tough after cooked.

**MUSHROOMS**: Mushrooms have a lot of liquid; before using them wipe the off with a damp towel to clean them and for storage place them in brown paper bag and they will last much longer.

**BROTHS**: Always make your broth in large quantities and store the remaining in the freezer. They will keep very well for up to 6 months. If you bake a chicken, save the carcass in a freezer bag and place in the freezer; add parts as they become available. Whenever I cook chicken I will put the wing tips, back or giblets in a freezer bag to use for making broth.

**MEATBALLS, HAMBURGER PATTIES AND MEATLOAF**: If you want to be sure your seasoned meat is right on point, cook a small amount of the seasoned meat in a frying pan and taste.

**PASTA**: Putting olive oil in your pasta water will keep the sauce from sticking to the pasta. If I plan on making a pasta salad the olive oil gives your pasta that sweet flavor and keeps it nice and loose.

**PASTA WATER**: When water comes to a boil, salt liberally, this will wake up the flavor of your pasta and it is the only opportunity to season your pasta.

**SEASON IN LAYERS**: Season and taste as you go and never serve your dish before tasting.

**BAKING POTATOES**: Preheat oven to $350^0$, wash and scrub potato skin and dry with a paper towel; with a fork, poke some holes in the potato skin, rub potato skin with canola oil and place on rack in the middle of the oven. Place a baking sheet on the shelf below to catch any drippings and bake for one hour. DO NOT WRAP IN FOIL, this way the potato skin will be nice and crisp.

**BACON FAT**: Keep a jar of reserve bacon fat in your refrigerator. It adds a nice smoky flavor to sautéed vegetables, gravies of other dishes. If you don't want to add bacon, but want the flavor, a little dab goes a long way.

**BACON SLICES**: Keeping some bacon in the freezer makes it easy to slice or chop.

# SAUCES

Since moving to North Carolina, I have discovered that I love to garden and once again my Aunt Mae influences my life. While growing up in Boston, she would take me and her Cocker Spaniel, Wendy, to her 10x10 public garden space behind Fenway Park.

One of the many items I grow in my garden are peppers; chili peppers, habaneros, jalapenos and of course, orange, red, yellow, green and sometime purple bell peppers.

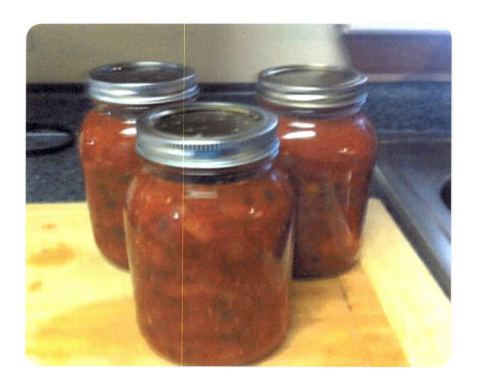

# 3 Pepper Hot Sauce

## INGREDIENTS:

2 Tablespoons Olive Oil

2 Habaneras – seeded & sliced

12 Jalapeños – seeded & sliced

20 Red Chili Peppers –seeded & sliced

1 whole onion (medium sized) diced

4 large garlic cloves – minced

6 fresh basil leaves – chopped

1 quart of whole tomatoes (I used canned tomatoes
   from my garden)

1 cup of white distilled vinegar

3 teaspoons of kosher salt

3 teaspoons of sugar

## DIRECTIONS:

Heat a medium size sauce pan and add olive oil, peppers, onion, garlic & sauté for 10 minutes to wake up those flavors. Then add tomatoes, vinegar, basil leaves, salt, pepper & sugar. Bring to a boil, lower heat and let simmer for 2 hours. In batches puree the mixture in blender –taste and if necessary, add salt, pepper, sugar or vinegar to your preference. You can store your hot sauce in the refrigerator for up to 3 months or in the freezer for up to 1 year. I often can my hot sauce if I make a large quantity it keeps for up to a year unopened.

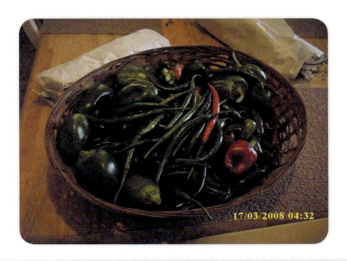

# Food items I like to keep on hand!

All Purpose Flour

Apple Cider Vinegar,

Balsamic Vinegar

White Wine Vinegar

Rice Vinegar

Champagne Vinegar

Red Wine Vinegar

White Vinegar (55% acidity)

Bell Peppers (diced in freezer)

Butter Milk

Brown Sugar

Mason Jars

Catsup – low fructose or my own awesome homemade catsup

Cheese Cloth

Confectioners' Sugar

Deli Meat – such as honey bake and maple ham, turkey and pastrami – all freeze well up to 3 months

Dried Mustard

Fresh Garlic

Fresh Ginger (store peeled whole, slices or grated in freezer)

*Fresh Herbs – parsley and cilantro are very all purpose herbs

Garlic Powder

Ginger Paste in a tube

Masala Wine

White Wine

Red Wine

Granulated Sugar

Grated and Shredded Parmesan Cheese – both freeze well up to 3 months

Half and Half

Honey

Hungarian Paprika

Kosher Salt

Liquid Smoke

Molasses

Mushrooms

Onion Powder

Pasta – a variety

Pepper Mill for freshly ground pepper

Ready to Use Seasonings (recipes follow)

Saffron Strands

San Marzano crushed tomatoes

San Marzano whole tomatoes

Smoked Paprika

Soy Sauce

**Steak Sauce

Sweet Onion

Tie String

Tomato Paste in a tube – keeps well in the refrigerator

Unsalted Butter

Virgin Coconut Oil

Worcestershire Sauce

Cayenne Pepper

Black Beans – canned and bags

Red Kidney Beans – canned and bags

Chick Peas – Canned and bags

Red Pepper Flakes (made from the pepper in my garden)

Yellow Onions

Ziploc Plastic Baggies – Small & Large – Frozen & Storage

*When I harvest my herb garden I dry or freeze and store them so I can always have fresh herbs on hand. You can always grow fresh herbs in your kitchen all year long!

**I like to make a big batch of steak sauce and either can it or place in the freezer – keeps for a year.

# My Favorite Herbs

There are 24 basic herbs, these are the ones that I grow in my herb garden and use frequently.

**BASIL - Sweet & spicy, licorice-like flavor.**

Other varieties: Purple basil, has a milder flavor, cinnamon basil, and lemon basil.

Tomatoes, zucchini, rice dishes, omelets, potato salad, macaroni salad and the main ingredient of pesto. I use purple basil to make red vinegar.

**BAY LEAVES - Also known as Laurel leaves - Savory.**

Great in soups and chowders; potatoes, pasta, spaghetti sauce, casseroles, beef and chicken stew, and in chicken and shrimp marinades. Always remove leaves when dish is done.

**CHIVES - Mild onion flavor.**

Great in quiche, spreads and dips, tuna salad, garden salad, potato salad, baked potatoes and practically all types of vegetables. Often used as a garnish for soups and many other dishes.

**CILANTRO - Citrus and sage flavor.**

Number one for Mexican dishes, salsa, tacos, chicken, fish, rice, pasta any type of vegetable dish. Makes a great butter for vegetables and fish and great for spicy dishes. Has a better and more intense flavor when used fresh instead of dried.

**DILL – Also known as dill weed.**

Great in bean soups; in egg dishes, and fish, especially salmon. Salad dressings, potato and macaroni salads and cabbage. Used for pickling cucumbers for kosher pickles.

**MARJORAM – Also known as sweet marjoram - Subtle lemon - more delicate than oregano**.

Great in pasta sauces; add great flavor to roasts, beef meatloaf, scrambled eggs and omelets; use with bread cubes for stuffing. Compliments green beans, mushrooms, carrots. Ideal for in stews, marinades, and herb butters

**MINT - Sweet-flavored, cool and refreshing.**

Great in summer drinks, on potatoes, green beans, and fruit salads, iced tea and lemonade; makes a beautiful garnish for desserts.

**OREGANO - Earthy and intense with a hint of clove**.

Great in any tomato dish; pasta sauces, pizza, chili, barbecue sauce. Excellent in egg and cheese dishes; meat or poultry stuffings; on pork, lamb, chicken and fish. Used in almost every Italian dish. This herb is better when dried.

**PARSLEY – This grows year round in North Carolina. It is very savory curly or flat leaf**.

Great in any pasta dish or Italian recipes; sauces, scrambled eggs, soups, mashed or boiled potatoes, all vegetable dishes, especially potatoes! Carrots, cabbage, tomatoes, turnip, beets; poultry or fish; soup or stew. Blends well with other herbs and is a beautiful garnish for potato or macaroni salad. I prefer fresh parsley to dried, this is easy to accomplish since it grows year round, stands up to frost.

**ROSEMARY – Grows year round, I use a lot of rosemary. It has a piney flavor with a hint of lemon; blends well with basil or thyme.**

Great with beef, pork, and poultry; when making a roast, make slits with a knife and insert garlic slivers and rosemary leaves. Use rosemary when cooking any type of squash and in sauce for lasagna; in vinegars, oils and marinades. I have added it to cornbread and biscuits. Rosemary is good fresh or dried.

**SAGE – Grows year round. Earthy and savory. Pineapple and purple sage are a bit milder**. Blends very well with rosemary, thyme or marjoram.

Great in stuffing for poultry; gives great flavor to fish, pork and beef; in sauces, soups, chowders and marinades; Add to barbecue sauces with rosemary and thyme. A strong herb so use sparingly. Deep fry sage leaves as an appetizer or garnish. Good with onions, cabbage, carrots, corn, squash, tomatoes and other vegetables. Make a sage butter for vegetables or pork.

**TARRAGON - Sweet, licorice – like flavor.**

Great in soups, with fish, any egg dish and garden salads. Add tarragon to vinegar for salad dressings; tartar sauce for salmon, or to make mayonnaise. Make a tarragon and lemon butter sauce and brush on grilled fish; excellent with chicken, pork, and beef; a main ingredient in Béarnaise sauce. Good with green beans, asparagus, peas or carrots. I use the yellow flowers along with the leaves for my tarragon vinegar.

**THYME – I never have enough Thyme! Very savory, Lemon thyme - a bit milder, with a lemony flavor.**
Blends well with other herbs especially rosemary.

Great with all meats, vegetables, casseroles, soups, stuffing, meatloaf, and marinades. Excellent for herb bread and flavored butters. Good with mushrooms, fried potatoes, carrots and all other vegetables; eggs and omelets. Fabulous in clam chowder and gumbo. Lemon thyme is great with fish and chicken. A strong herb even dried.

# Herbs That Compliment
## BEEF, PORK & POULTRY

**BEEF:**

Basil - Bay Leaf – Cumin – Fennell – Oregano – Parsley - Rosemary
Tarragon – Sage – Thyme


**PORK:**

Cumin –Curry – Ginger – Rosemary – Sage – Tarragon – Thyme - Turmeric


**POULTRY:**

Basil – Cardammon – Cumin – Fenell – Ginger – Marjoram -Tumeric
Nutmeg – Oregano – Parsley – Rosemary – Sage – Tarragon - Thyme

# Herbs and Vegetables

**<u>Asparagus</u>** - Dill, marjoram, nutmeg, rosemary

**<u>Broccoli</u>** - Garlic, marjoram, nutmeg

**<u>Brussels Sprouts</u>** - Rosemary, parsley, caraway, nutmeg, oregano, marjoram

**<u>Cabbage</u>** - Bay leaves, garlic, curry, marjoram, nutmeg, chives, parsley

**<u>Carrots</u>** - Parsley, basil, curry, chives, sage, thyme

**<u>Cauliflower</u>** - Basil, dill, mace, ginger, curry, nutmeg, oregano, coriander, mint

**<u>Cucumber</u>** - Rosemary, dill, mustard seed, pepper, basil, chives

**<u>Green Beans</u>** - Garlic, basil, dill, nutmeg, pepper

**<u>Leeks</u>** - Mustard, parsley, dill, bay leaves, thyme, paprika, celery seed

**<u>Lettuce</u>** - Basil, chives, thyme, tarragon, dill, parsley

**<u>Mushrooms</u>** - Olives, ginger, cumin, parsley, thyme

**Onions** - Smoked Paprika, celery salt, pepper, coriander, basil, garlic, marjoram, sage, tarragon, dill, rosemary

**<u>Peas</u>** - Tarragon, mint, parsley, nutmeg, sage, marjoram, basil

**<u>Potatoes</u>** - Garlic, nutmeg, paprika, pepper, rosemary, thyme

**<u>Tomatoes</u>** - Basil, tarragon, garlic, chives, dill, mint, oregano, paprika, fennel, parsley, thyme, curry

**<u>Zucchini</u>** - Garlic, basil, parsley, oregano, dill, rosemary

# HERBED VINEGARS & INFUSED OILS
## – Great for salads, fish and vegetables

### Tarragon Vinegar

1 cup tarragon leaves + 3 additional sprigs
2 cups white wine vinegar

**DIRECTIONS:**

Cut fresh green tarragon stems from the garden, wash and place on paper towel and pat dry. Remove leaves from stems and place in a sterile jar. Add the vinegar. Cover and store in a cool dark place for 2-3 weeks to let the tarragon infuse the vinegar. Strain vinegar and discard tarragon. In a separate sterilize bottle, add additional tarragon sprigs and vinegar.

Vinegar will keep for up to 6 months in cool dark place.

### Basil Vinegar

Made with sweet basil leaves, the same way as Tarragon Vinegar.
Use about 4 basil leaves for bottle garnish.

# Mixed Herb Vinegar

2 cup of parsley leaves + 1 sprig of parsley

1 cup basil leaves – 1 Floweret of Basil

6 whole garlic cloves

24 sprigs of chives

Red wine vinegar

**DIRECTIONS:**

Place all the herbs in a sterilized 16 oz. mason jar, fill with vinegar. Cover and store in cool dark place for 4 weeks. Strain vinegar and discard herbs. Place parsley sprig & basil in vinegar bottle and add vinegar. Cover tightly and keep in cool dry place. Good for up to 6 months.

# Garlic Infused Olive Oil

1 cup of very good extra virgin olive oil

8 cloves of garlic – thinly sliced

**DIRECTIONS:**

Heat oil in saucepan, remove from heat and add garlic slices. Let sit until cooled; remove garlic, strain through cheesecloth if necessary. Place oil in nice bottle and use for cooking or for salads.

# Italian Blend Olive Oil

2 cups of very good extra virgin olive oil

4 medium sprigs of oregano + 1 sprig for garnish

6 sprigs of fresh thyme + 1 sprig for garnish

10 large fresh sweet basil leaves + 1 large leaf for
garnish

4 garlic cloves

1 teaspoon of Kosher Salt

## DIRECTIONS:

Heat oil in saucepan, remove from heat and add herbs. Place in glass or plastic bowl, cover with cellophane and let sit for 24 hours.

In a nice bottle, add salt, garlic, basil leaf, 1 sprig each or thyme and oregano, and then add infused olive oil. Use to sauté vegetables for spaghetti or marinara sauce or add red wine vinegar for an Italian Dressing for salads or to brush on bread and pizza dough for homemade pizza.

## Garlic Fused Olive Oil

Roasted Garlic Bulb
Kosher Salt
Extra Virgin Oil

## DIRECTIONS:

To roast your garlic: Cut the top off of a garlic bulb. Place on a piece of foil and pour about 1 teaspoon of olive oil over the top and rub in the oil all over the top and sides. Close the foil and roast in oven at 400⁰ for about 30 minutes. Remove from oven and let cool until you are able to squeeze out the garlic. In a 8 ounce Mason Jar (or other airtight glass container), add 1 tablespoon of Kosher Salt (preservative), add the garlic and cover with the olive oil. Store in a cool dark place and it will keep for 3 months. Mine never lasts that long because I use it often.

## USES:

Garlic Bread: Brush on and broil
To sauté vegetables
Steaks
Any use that you want to use a garlic flavored olive oil….let your imagination soar!

# Seasonings, Rubs, Sauces and Brines

Keep these spice mixtures on hand for convenience; they can be used to season meat, as rubs or marinades. By making your own, you can control the salt intake and avoid any preservatives. You can double or even triple these recipes for storage. My preference for storage containers are Mason Jars, but air tight containers or even Ziploc bags work just as well; always store away from direct light. I have found that about 3 tablespoons to 1lb of meat is a fair ratio; however, feel free to use more or less, to your preference.

## All Purpose Poultry Seasonings

3 tablespoons of Hungarian Paprika

2 tablespoons of thyme

2 tablespoons of sage

2 tablespoons of rosemary

1 teaspoon kosher salt

2 tablespoons of course black pepper

Mix until well combined

## All Purpose Pork Seasoning

2 tablespoons of kosher salt

2 tablespoons of coarsely ground black pepper

1 teaspoon of curry powder

½ teaspoon of turmeric

2 tablespoons of dried rosemary

1 teaspoon ground yellow mustard

Mix until well combined

## All Purpose Beef Seasonings

2 tablespoons of kosher salt

2 tablespoons of coarsely ground black pepper

2 tablespoons of rosemary

3 tablespoons of garlic powder

2 tablespoons of onion powder

2 tablespoons of thyme

## Chili Seasonings

2 tablespoons of all-purpose flour

3 tablespoons garlic powder

3 tablespoons of onion powder

2 tablespoons of dark brown sugar

½ cup of ground cumin*

4 tablespoons dried parsley

3 tablespoons dried basil

4 tablespoons of coarsely ground black pepper

2 tablespoons kosher salt

3 tablespoons smoked paprika

2 tablespoons cayenne pepper

2 tablespoons of chipotle chili powder

NOTE: For more heat add more cayenne pepper

*For a more intense flavor you can toast 1 cup of cumin seeds on medium heat until they become fragrant. Stir constantly to avoid burning seeds. When toasted crush in mortar or in coffee bean grinder

# RUBS:

For oven roasting, frying or on the grill, rubs are a great way to get the spices right in the meat. Not only will you get a great flavor, but your meat will stay nice & moist. For an even more intense flavor, rub your meat the night before, wrap tightly in plastic wrap and store on the bottom shelf of your refrigerator. If time does not allow you to let your meat sit over night, I recommend at least 4 hours, of course you can always rub and cook. You can also freeze your meat after it has been rubbed. Rub the meat thoroughly, wrap tightly in plastic wrap, and then place in freezer bag. It will keep for up to a month. When ready to prepare, let meat thaw in the refrigerator and do your thing. For a wet rub, just add about 1 -2 tablespoons of olive oil, lemon juice or vinegar.

## Barbeque Rib - Rub

1 tablespoon of kosher salt

2 tablespoons of smoked paprika

2 tablespoons of garlic powder

2 tablespoons of onion powder

5 finely chopped sage leaves

2 sprigs thyme leaves

2 tablespoons of brown sugar (optional)*

2 tablespoons of course black pepper

1 tablespoon of crushed red pepper

Pinch of ground nutmeg

*brown sugar adds a great flavor when grilling

Mix well.

Double or triple the recipe and reserve in an air tight container. Stays flavorful for up to 6 months.

## Poultry Rub

2 tablespoons of dried thyme

1 tablespoon kosher salt:

2 tablespoons of course ground pepper

3 tablespoons of coffee grinds

1 tablespoons of garlic powder

1 tablespoons of onion powder

Blend well – rinse poultry in cool water and dry with paper towel. Cover poultry with rub, place on plate and put in refrigerator (uncover) on the bottom shelf for at least 2 hours or overnight.

## Coffee Grind Rub

1 cup coffee grinds

4 tablespoons kosher salt

2 tablespoons coarse black pepper

### DIRECTIONS:

Rub coffee grinds on washed and dried chicken, place in refrigerator uncover overnight uncovered. Before grilling or bake in oven –drizzle with extra virgin olive oil.

Great on chicken, beef and fish.

## Pork Rub

4 tablespoons of smoked paprika

2 teaspoons of curry powder

1 teaspoon of ground ginger

2 tablespoons of garlic powder

2 tablespoons of onion powder

2 tablespoons of brown sugar

1 teaspoon chili powder

2 tablespoons of finely chopped rosemary (2 sprigs)

1 teaspoon of allspice (optional)

**Keep your rubs in air tight jars, of course I use Mason jars. Store away from direct light and they will keep for at least 6 months.**

# BARBEQUE SAUCES

## PORK RIBS – Barbeque Sauce

### INGREDIENTS:

2 tablespoons of extra virgin olive oil

1 ½ finely chopped Spanish onions

3 minced garlic cloves

2 cups of catsup – fructose free (or use your own fabulous homemade catsup)

1 cup of water

½ cup of brown sugar

¼ cup of granulated white sugar

1 ½ teaspoons of ground black pepper

1 teaspoon of kosher salt

½ cup of apple cider vinegar

Juice of 1 lemon – after juicing lemon cut up in slices to add to sauce

3 tablespoons of Pork Rub

1 sprig of rosemary leaves – finely chopped

### DIRECTIONS:

In saucepan add olive oil, add onion & garlic and cook for 5 – 8 minutes or until tender. Add catsup, water, brown & white sugar, pepper, salt, vinegar, lemon juice, lemon slices and pork rub, mix well. Bring to boil and simmer for 1 hour. Remove lemon slices.

# POULTRY – Barbecue Sauce

## INGREDIENTS:

2 tablespoons of extra virgin olive oil

1 ½ finely chopped Spanish onions

3 minced garlic cloves

2 cups of catsup – fructose free

½ cup of water

1 cup of honey

1 ½ teaspoons of ground black pepper

1 teaspoon of kosher salt

Juice of 2 lemons – after juicing lemon cut up in
    slices to add to sauce

1 Bay Leaf

3 tablespoons of Poultry Rub – see recipe on
    page 16

5 finely chopped sage leaves

2 sprigs of thyme leaves

## DIRECTIONS:

In saucepan add olive oil, add onion & garlic and cook for 5 – 8 minutes or until tender. Add catsup, water, honey, pepper, salt, lemon juice, lemon slices and poultry rub, mix well. Bring to boil and simmer for 1 hour. Remove lemon slices and bay leaf. Add sage & thyme mix well.

Always taste your recipe

# Awesome-All Purpose Barbeque Sauce

## INGREDIENTS:

2 cups of Ketchup

2 cups of chicken broth

5 tablespoon dark brown sugar

2 tablespoons soy sauce

½ cup honey

½ cup dark molasses

3 tablespoons of Dijon mustard

Juice of 1 lime

1-12oz can of tomato paste

2 teaspoons of liquid smoke

¼ cup Worcestershire Sauce

3 minced garlic cloves - minced

1 cup finely chopped onions

1 tablespoon ground black pepper

½ teaspoon cayenne pepper

## DIRECTIONS:

Combine all ingredients in a large saucepan over a low heat. Stirring occasionally, bring to a boil and let simmer for 45-60 minutes, sauce should start to thicken. Allow to cool. Puree in blender or use an immersion blender. Store in an air tight container or a Mason jar and refrigerate. Sauce is best when it is allowed to sit for a day before using.

These sauces will keep in your refrigerator for 4 weeks always label with expiration date.

You can also store in the freezer for up to 6 months.

# Quick and Easy Spaghetti Sauce

## INGREDIENTS:

2 (28 oz.) cans crushed tomatoes

1 small can of tomato paste

1 large onion – diced

1 large green pepper – diced

3-4 cloves of garlic – crushed

1 tablespoon of dried oregano

1 tablespoon of dried basil

Extra Virgin Olive Oil

1-2 tablespoons of brown sugar

½ teaspoon crushed red pepper

½ each of salt & pepper (to taste)

## DIRECTIONS:

In Dutch oven or large saucepan add EVOO to cover bottom of pan. Add onion, green pepper, garlic and sauté 5-8 minutes; add oregano & basil stir to coat vegetables. Add tomatoes, paste, sugar salt & pepper and let simmer 30-45 minutes.

Serve as is or purée.

*Always taste your recipe during and after preparation.*

*These sauces will keep in your refrigerator for 4 weeks.*

*If storing in refrigerator, label with expiration date.*

*You can also store in the freezer for up to 6 months.*

# Hearty Spaghetti Sauce

My favorite cousin, who lives in Upstate New York, asked me for my spaghetti recipe, although, I already had one, I was inspired to create a more "hearty" recipe. When she asked me for the recipe New York was getting hammered with snow and freezing temperatures. There are 3 meats and lots of vegetables and time to spend in your kitchen on a cold winter's day. Read through the recipe and be sure you have all the ingredients you need. Prepare by chopping, mincing and dicing all your vegetables and placing in them in containers for easy accessibility. Chop and mix your herbs and place them in small bowls or cups and have your spices at hand so they will be ready for you when you are ready for them.

## INGREDIENTS for MEATBALLS:

2 lbs. chopped sirloin – for meatballs

1 large onion – finely chopped

4 garlic cloves minced

2 tablespoons dried oregano

2 tablespoons dried thyme

½ cup chopped fresh parsley

1 tablespoon kosher salt

2 tablespoons coarse black pepper

3 tablespoon mayo

2 tablespoons Dijon mustard

2 tablespoons extra virgin olive oil

3 large eggs – beaten

1 cup of Italian breadcrumbs

½ cup grated parmesan cheese

Extra Virgin Olive Oil

## DIRECTIONS FOR MEATBALLS

PREHEAT OVEN TO 350⁰. Combine chopped sirloin and all of the first ingredients in a large bowl and mix until well combined. Make small meatballs using a small ice cream scoop or teaspoon. Lightly coat 2 cookie sheets with olive oil, place meatballs on cookie sheet and bake for 10 minutes or until brown and set aside.

## INGREDIENTS:

6 ITALIAN SAUSAGES

## SAUSAGE – DIRECTIONS:

Place sausages on a lightly oiled baking dish and bake at 350⁰ for 15-20 minutes, until browned – let cool, slice and set aside.

## INGREDIENTS FOR THE SAUCE:

3 tablespoons of extra virgin olive oil

1 lb. ground pork

1 red bell pepper diced

1 yellow bell pepper diced

1 orange bell pepper diced

2 medium sweet onions diced

1 lb. of portabella mushrooms – thinly sliced

4 garlic cloves – minced

1 teaspoon ground cinnamon

1/8 teaspoon ground nutmeg

¼ cup of brown sugar

3 tablespoons kosher salt - divided

3 tablespoons coarse black pepper - divided

½ teaspoon crushed red pepper

1-6 oz can tomato paste

2-28 oz. cans of crushed tomatoes

1-Qt jar of your seeded canned tomatoes or 1-28 oz. can of whole plum tomatoes

¼ cup freshly chopped oregano

¼ cup freshly chopped basil leaves

10 sprigs of thyme – leaves removed and chopped

1 teaspoon freshly chopped rosemary

1/8 teaspoon fennel seeds – crushed

## The SAUCE- DIRECTIONS:

In medium sized stock pot heat extra virgin olive oil, add pork, peppers, onions, garlic, fennel seeds, and 2 tablespoons each of salt & pepper and cook until meat is brown. Mix in tomato paste and cook for another 3 minutes, stirring constantly until well blended. Add crushed tomatoes, whole tomatoes and juice, mushrooms, cinnamon, nutmeg, brown sugar, crushed pepper, bring to a boil and let simmer for 1 hour, stirring occasionally. Add herbs, meatballs, sausages and let simmer another 45 minutes.

Serve with your favorite spaghetti or pasta with a nice bruschetta or garlic and herb bread and a simple salad.

# Steak Sauce

I found several steak sauce recipes and after trial and error these are the ingredients that helped me make "the perfect" steak sauce. Make a batch and can it!

## INGREDIENTS:

12 Plum tomatoes diced or 2 – 28 ounce cans of diced

2 cups beef or vegetable stock

1 tablespoons of Extra Virgin Olive Oil

1 large Vidalia or sweet onion

1 cup of ketchup (fructose free – or homemade)

1 jalapeno pepper, seeded and minced

6 garlic cloves - chopped

½ cup light brown sugar

¼ cup freshly squeezed orange juice

Juice of 1 freshly squeezed lemon

2 tablespoons rice wine vinegar

2 tablespoons apple cider vinegar

3 tablespoon dark molasses

¼ cup of Worcestershire sauce

Medium size knob of minced fresh ginger

1/4 - 2 teaspoons chili powder

1 tablespoon cayenne – or less if you do not want too spicy or more if you like it HOT

½ tablespoon of kosher salt (or to taste)

1 tablespoon coarse black pepper

1/8 teaspoon nutmeg

## DIRECTIONS:

In medium to large stock pot heat olive, add garlic, onion, jalapeno, ginger, tomatoes, chili powder and cayenne pepper, salt and pepper and sauté for about 5-10 minutes or until vegetables are soft and fragrant. Stir in stock, brown sugar, nutmeg, orange & lemon juices, vinegars, molasses, Worcestershire sauce, ketchup, and cook to a boil. Reduce heat and let simmer for 1 hour.

Remove sauce from the heat and puree in blender or use immersion blender.

Put back in pot and taste for preferences, let simmer for another ½ hour.

# BARBEQUE SAUCE

## Barbeque Sauce for PORK RIBS

2 tablespoons of extra virgin olive oil

1 ½ finely chopped Spanish onions

3 minced garlic cloves

2 cups of catsup – fructose free (or use your own
    fabulous homemade catsup)

1 cup of water

½ cup of brown sugar

¼ cup of granulated white sugar

1 ½ teaspoons of ground black pepper

1 teaspoon of kosher salt

½ cup of apple cider vinegar

Juice of 1 lemon – after juicing lemon cut up in
    slices to add to sauce

3 tablespoons of Pork Rub

1 sprig of rosemary leaves – finely chopped

**DIRECTIONS**:

In saucepan add olive oil, add onion & garlic and cook for 5 – 8 minutes or until tender. Add catsup, water, brown & white sugar, pepper, salt, vinegar, lemon juice, lemon slices and pork rub, mix well. Bring to boil and simmer for 1 hour. Remove lemon slices.

# Barbeque Sauce for Poultry

2 tablespoons of extra virgin olive oil

1 ½ finely chopped Spanish onions

3 minced garlic cloves

2 cups of catsup – fructose free

½ cup of water

1 cup of honey

1 ½ teaspoons of ground black pepper

1 teaspoon of kosher salt

Juice of 2 lemons – after juicing lemon cut up in slices to add to sauce

3 tablespoons of Poultry Rub

5 finely chopped sage leaves

2 sprigs of thyme leaves

**DIRECTIONS**:

In saucepan add olive oil, add onion & garlic and cook for 5 – 8 minutes or until tender. Add catsup, water, honey, pepper, salt, lemon juice, lemon slices and poultry rub, mix well. Bring to boil and simmer for 1 hour. Remove lemon slices and bay leaf. Add sage & thyme mix well.

# IT'S BRINE TIME

I seldom cook any meat or poultry without brining. Brining keeps the meat or poultry tender, juicy and adds flavor. I find the ideal amount of time to brine is over night, if this is not possible I suggest at least 1 hour per pound to get the full benefits of your brine, or you can always "RUB IT."

Then I add ingredients according to what I am brining and how it will be prepared. You want to place your brining ingredients in stock pot large enough so your meat or poultry is completely immersed in the brining solution.

When brining is complete rinse your meat or poultry under cold water, then prepare as desired. If you want your poultry to roast with a nice golden brown skin; after you rinse the bird, pat dry and place uncovered in the refrigerator for at least 3 hours or until completely dry.

## POULTRY BRINE:

Fill stock pot with:

½ to 1 cup Kosher Salt

Water – enough to cover the meat

1 cup Brown Sugar

Sliced Lemon(s)/Sliced Orange(s)

2-6 springs of Rosemary

20 Sage Leaves

4-8 springs of Fresh Thyme

1 whole onion sliced in ½

½ to 1 whole garlic bulb cut in half

ICE

## <u>DIRECTIONS</u>:

Bring water and ingredients to a low boil and stir until salt & sugars have dissolved. Add 1 – 2 cups of ice to cool down. DO NOT ADD MEAT OR POULTRY TO HOT BRINE; bring it to room temperature or cooler (you do not want to cook your meat). Let meat brine for at least 4 hours or overnight.

**I brine my Thanksgiving turkey Tuesday to Thursday**

## **PORK CHOPS**:

4 cups of water, ¼ cup of sugar, ½ cup of brown sugar

When brining add different flavors, such as, peppercorns, preserved lemons, tarragon, mustard seeds, apples, oranges, limes or oregano or spice it up with chili or jalapeno peppers.

# Poultry Brine with Lemon and Thyme

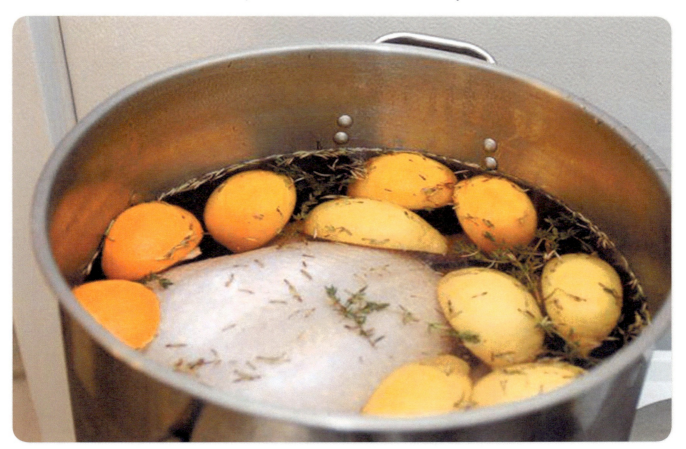

# POULTRY

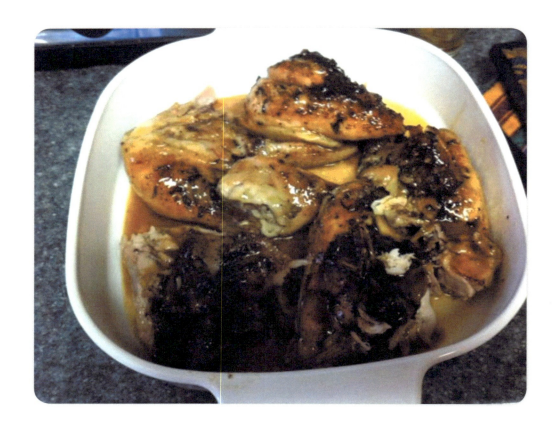

**Honey – Lemon Tarragon Baked Chicken**

# Honey - Lemon Chicken with Tarragon

**INGREDIENTS**:

6-8 Chicken parts – wings and legs

1 lemon divided – ½ juiced – ½ thinly sliced

2 teaspoons kosher salt

1 tablespoon of freshly ground or course black
   pepper

3 garlic cloves minced

¼ cup extra virgin olive oil

1 cup of pure honey

1 ½ tablespoons of dried Tarragon

Marinade chicken overnight or at least 4 hours

**DIRECTIONS:**

Marinade:

Mix lemon juice, garlic, and olive oil in a small bowl.

Rinse chicken under cold water, pat dry with paper towel, season with salt and pepper, place in plastic Ziploc bag, pour marinade in bag, seal and place in refrigerator on a plate on the bottom shelf of refrigerator.

PREHEAT OVEN 350⁰

Remove chicken from marinate (discard marinade); place chicken in small roasting pan that has a cover or baking dish. Sprinkle with tarragon, lay lemon slices on top then add the honey. Cover pan and place in oven for 45 minutes; baste chicken, place back in oven without cover and bake another 15 – 20 minutes, until chicken is done.

# Angel's Shake and Baked Chicken Breasts

PREHEAT OVEN TO: 450º

4 – 6 chicken breast – bone in

1 cup of all-purpose flour

1.5 teaspoons of kosher salt

2 tablespoons course black pepper

2 teaspoons of smoked paprika

1 teaspoon of ground sage

1 tablespoons of ground thyme

1 stick of unsalted butter

2 tablespoons of freshly chopped parsley for garnish

**<u>DIRECTIONS</u>**:

Mix flour, salt & pepper, paprika, sage, and thyme in a bag. Add chicken breast and shake until well coated. Melt butter in oven in a medium sized baking dish. Place chicken, skin side down in baking dish and bake for 20 – 25 minutes, then turn and bake on the other side for 20-25 minutes or until done and juices are running clear. Remove from oven and place in serving dish, cover with foil and let sit 5 minutes before serving.

Light Sauce – Optional: Remove drippings to small sauce pan, add about 2 tablespoons of butter (if necessary), stir in 2 tablespoons of all purpose flour and whisk well (about 2 minutes) add about 1 cup of chicken broth and continue to whisk, add more broth if necessary to your desired consistency. Add ½ teaspoon of sage, ½ teaspoon of thyme them salt & pepper to taste

FOR A BIT MORE RICHNESS, SUBSTITUTE THE CHICKEN BROTH FOR A NICE WHITE WINE…yum!

Pour sauce directly over chicken and garnish with parsley or serve on the side.

# Boneless Stuffed Chicken Thighs

**<u>INGREDIENTS</u>:**

6 Boneless Chicken Thighs

4 garlic cloves, sliced

¼ cup extra virgin olive oil

1 lime – juiced and zested

1 teaspoon kosher salt

2 teaspoons course black pepper

2 tablespoons dried Thyme

4 tablespoons fresh cilantro - chopped

2 teaspoons dried cumin

1 teaspoon Salt

2 teaspoons coarse black Pepper

1 bags of baby spinach

1 lb. portabella mushrooms

3 jalapeños – halved, seeded, ribs removed – thinly sliced

6 Smoked ham slices

1 cup plain Panko bread crumbs

Butter

3 eggs beaten for breading of chicken

Toothpicks – 6 or more

2 cups of all-purpose flour

Marinade: – Garlic, olive oil, lime, salt & pepper, cilantro, thyme & cumin. Place chicken in Ziploc bag with marinade, place in refrigerator for at least 4 hours or overnight.

Preheat Oven to 350⁰

**<u>DIRECTIONS</u>:**

In sauté pan melt 2 tables of butter, add mushrooms, jalapeños and spinach and cook until spinach wilts and set aside. Butter a casserole dish large enough for the 6 chicken breasts.

Prepare breading station – place bread crumbs in a plate, beat 3 in a medium bowl and another bowl for the flour.

Lightly salt & pepper the chicken thighs on both sides. Place a slice of ham inside the chicken thigh, add the mushroom mixture, and roll tightly tucking in the ends so the mixture does not fall out. Roll thighs in flour, then egg mixture and roll in breadcrumbs, hold together with toothpick(s) and place in casserole dish.

Place chicken in oven and bake for 45 minutes until chicken is tender.

# PRESERVED LEMONS

Preserved lemons add a deliciously pungent flavor to chicken, fish, rice and vegetables. There are a lot a different ways to preserve lemons. This is how I do it:

I like to use small lemons or if you can get them Meyers Lemons.

**<u>DIRECTIONS</u>**:
Wash and scrub your whole lemons and wipe dry. Slice into quarters. In a glass or ceramic dish lay quarters in one layer, skin side down and sprinkle liberally with kosher salt until all the lemons are cover. Then pack tightly in a sterilized Mason jar and fill with lemon juice. Cover and place on table or counter top upside down for 2 days, then flip right side up for two days. Store in a cool dark cabinet until ready to use. An unopened jar will be good for up to 1 year, however, after opening, place in the refrigerator. They will last a long time – but my mine never does, because I use them often.

**<u>Variations</u>**:
You can add a few bays leaves, some cloves or even garlic or jalapenos.

# Butterfly Roasted Chicken with Preserved Lemon

We have said, in my household, that we eat so much chicken one day we will grow wings. There are just so many recipes for poultry. You can bake it, fry it, boil it, barbeque it, sauté it; make soup, salad and sandwiches. You can add almost any type of flavor from peppered chicken to honey chicken. Well this is one of many "Lemon-Chicken" recipes you will discover in my cookbook, because lemon and chicken were made for each other.

Butterflying a chicken cuts down on cooking time so this makes a great weeknight meal!

Brine the chicken the night before!

PREHEAT OVEN TO 400⁰

### INGREDIENTS:

1 whole roasting chicken

Olive Oil

1 garlic bulb – cloves separated, smashed and paper removed

Kosher Salt

Coarse Black Pepper

6 wedges of preserved lemon (pulp removed) skin thinly sliced

6 sprigs of fresh Rosemary

1 carrot cut in quarters

1 celery stalk cut in quarters

1 onion cut in quarters

Hungarian Paprika

6 tablespoons of softened unsalted butter

### BUTTERFLY YOUR CHICKEN:

Rinse chicken thoroughly and pat dry with paper towels. Place on your "meat" cutting board with the breast side down and the neck cavity facing you. Cut along back bone on both sides to remove.* Turn the chicken over and press down on the breastbone to break it. Voila, a butterflied chicken.

## **DIRECTIONS**:

Coat the bottom of a large roasting pan with olive oil. On your "meat only" cutting board generously salt & pepper your chicken on both sides. Place your chicken in roasting pan breast side up. Under the chicken (in the cavity) place your carrot, celery and onion, then spread your garlic, lemon and Rosemary on top and around the chicken and generously cover with olive oil and sprinkle with paprika.

Bake uncovered for 35 minutes, remove from oven and slather with butter (this will make the skin a golden brown), return to oven for another 10 minutes – until done.

This goes great with garlic smashed potatoes and roasted Brussels sprouts.

# BEEF KABOBS on the GRILL with Preserved Lemons

## INGREDIENTS:

1 lb beef tenderloin - trimmed and cubed into 8 pieces

1 red bell pepper- seeded- diced large

1 green bell pepper- seeded- diced large

8 preserved lemon wedges-rinsed-pulp removed

1 red onion- diced large

2 tablespoons chopped fresh parsley leaves

3 chopped garlic cloves

2 teaspoons dried oregano

2 teaspoons onion powder

1 teaspoon curry powder

1 teaspoon Turmeric

1 tablespoon kosher salt

2 teaspoons fresh ground black pepper

1 cup extra virgin olive oil

4 skewers- if you are using wood soak them in water for 30 minutes to keep them from burning

## DIRECTIONS:

Prepare your meat and vegetables by cleaning, seeding, cubing and chopping and set aside.

Thread a piece of green pepper, a cube of beef, preserved lemon wedge, couple of pieces of red onion, another piece of beef, red pepper and top it with a mushroom. Repeat with the rest of the skewers. Place kabobs in a roasting pan in one layer and set aside. In medium size bowl add: parsley, garlic oregano, onion & curry powder, Turmeric, salt, pepper and olive oil and mix well. Pour over kabobs and marinate in refrigerator at least one hour or overnight.

Preheat an outdoor charcoal or gas grill to high heat or top stove grill. Place the kabobs on the grill and cook about 3 - 5 minutes per side, depending on your preference. Remove and let sit for about 2 minutes before serving.

You may also prepare these in the oven. Place on a rack on a baking sheet and cook at 350º for 20 minutes or until beef is at your liking and the vegetables are done, but still crisp.

# Boneless Chicken Thighs with Preserved Lemons

## INGREDIENTS:

2 tablespoons canola oil

4 chicken thigh boneless – skinned

2- 4 garlic cloves minced

1 teaspoon fresh gingerroot, chopped

1/2 teaspoon cayenne pepper

1/2 teaspoon paprika

½ cup vegetable stock

Juice of 1 lemon

2 quarters preserved lemons- rinsed-pulp removed-
  sliced in thin slivers

1 tablespoon chopped fresh parsley

## DIRECTIONS:

Place oil in heavy frying pan and brown chicken over high heat on all sides. Remove from the pan and set aside. Place the onion, garlic and ginger in a food processor and work until smooth.

Add puree to the frying pan and stir over medium heat for a minute, add the cayenne pepper, paprika, lemon juice and stock. Stir to combine and bring to a boil. Lower the heat and simmer for 5-8 minutes. Add chicken, lemon slivers and cook further for 15 minutes – until chicken is done. Sprinkle with parsley and serve over Jasmine Rice.

# Salmon Salad with Preserved Lemons

**INGREDIENTS:**

2 tablespoons olive oil

2 - 4 garlic clove

3 quarters preserved lemon – rinsed-pulp removed
    cut into thin slivers

1 ½ cups of pasta (whatever your preference)

1 cup Snow Peas

2 -salmon steaks, skin removed

Salt and pepper

1 bunch Dill leaves tops finely chopped

1 tablespoon of infused garlic olive oil

**DIRECTIONS:**

Heat 1 tablespoon olive oil in frying pan and add garlic to fuse the oil over medium high heat, until the garlic is fragrant, do not let it BURN! Remove the garlic and set it aside.

THE PASTA: Cook pasta according to the directions, add the Snow Peas about 3 minutes before pasta is done. Then drain; place in bowl and add the lemon, dill and olive oil and Salt & Pepper to taste and toss. Cover and set aside.

***THE SALMON***: Brush salmon with olive oil on both sides; add salt & pepper to taste place in frying pan with the infused garlic oil over medium to high heat. Cook 4 -8 minutes each side depending on your preference. Let cool for about 5 minutes then flake with a fork. Add to Pasta Mixture and toss. Garnish with fresh dill leaves.

# Chicken Pesto Roll Ups with a Luscious-Light Sauce

PREHEAT OVEN TO 375⁰

**INGREDIENTS**:

3 Boneless-Skinless Chicken Breasts – cut in
   halves – pound* to about a ¼ inch thick

Salt & Pepper

1 cup of Lemon-Basil Pesto

Toothpicks

2 eggs beaten

2 cups of all-purpose flour + 4 tablespoons for sauce

2 cups Italian seasoned panko bread crumbs

6 tablespoons of unsalted butter

1 cup good white wine – preferably Riesling

**DIRECTIONS**:

Melt butter in oven-proof glass baking dish – remove and set aside. Prepare breading station. Lightly salt & pepper chicken breasts and spread 2 tablespoons of pesto on each breast, roll up and secure with toothpicks to prevent pesto from escaping. Then dip each roll up in flour, then egg, then panko. Place in baking dish and cook for 50 until done.

Remove chicken to serving dish and cover with foil. Save dripping for Sauce.

Luscious – Light Sauce: Pour and scrape juices and brown goodness from the baking dish into a small sauce pan onto medium-low heat if necessary add more butter. Add flour and stir until you form your roux. Add 2 tablespoon (or remaining) pesto, mix well. Add wine to preferred consistency, add salt & pepper if necessary. Pour sauce over chicken and serve.

*Place chicken between two pieces of wax paper or cellophane and pound with a meat mallet to desired thinness. Be careful not to tear the breasts or make too thin.

# Creamed Chicken with Mushrooms

## INGREDIENTS:

6 – 10 Chicken parts – wings, legs and thighs

1 tablespoon of kosher salt

2 tablespoons freshly ground or course black pepper

2 tablespoons of smoked paprika

1/3 cup flour + 2 tablespoons - divided

½ stick unsalted butter + 2 tablespoons

4 tablespoons + 1 tablespoon of Extra Virgin Olive Oil - divided

2 cups of sliced baby portabella mushrooms – about 12 -15 mushrooms

2 garlic cloves – minced

½ large or 1 small onion - sliced

1 cup vegetable broth

1 cup of fat free half and half

½ teaspoon ground marjoram

½ teaspoon of ground sage

## DIRECTIONS:

Season chicken with salt, pepper and paprika, put flour in plastic bag, add chicken and shake bag to coat lightly coat chicken with flour.

In 12" sauté pan, add ½ stick of butter and 4 tablespoons of olive oil, brown chicken on all sides, remove to plate lined with paper towels and set aside. Pour oil from pan, (do not wash pain) return pan to a medium flame add 2 tablespoons butter, 1 teaspoon olive oil when butter melts, add mushrooms, onions, garlic, salt, pepper, marjoram, sage, sauté until mushrooms are nice and brown, about 5 – 8 minutes. Add 3 tablespoons of flour, and stir with vegetables until well blended then add broth and half & half, mix well, bring to boil. Return chicken to pan, lower heat and let simmer for 45 minutes to 1 hour. Stir and baste occasionally. Place in serving dish and garnish with freshly chopped parsley.

Meal: Serve with white or brown rice and your favorite vegetable…something green.

*Growing your own herbs is not only rewarding, but it inspires you to create ways to utilize them. Rosemary is strong, yet beautifully fragrant herb, so you have to be careful not to use too much, but it gives chicken such a wonderful flavor. Just sniff it and you will be inspired too. Rosemary & chicken, what a great combo!*

# Rosemary-Roasted Chicken with Potatoes and Carrots

Preheat oven to or roaster to 350° Fahrenheit

**INGREDIENTS**:

1 Whole Chicken cut in parts

Kosher salt & freshly ground black pepper

1 Ziploc baggie

1 cup and 3 tablespoons of all-purpose flour

2 tablespoons of smoked paprika

4 sprigs of fresh Rosemary – divided

1½ cups canola oil

Extra Virgin Olive Oil

6 large fresh Sage leaves – finely chopped

1 large onion – diced

4 large carrots –sliced (diagonal)

4 russet potatoes – cut in 2 inch cubes

1 celery stalk – 1 inch slices

4 – 6 garlic cloves – finely chopped

1 cup of chicken broth

**DIRECTIONS**:

Prep: Cut up potatoes, carrots, garlic, celery, & sage leaves, place in bowl and set aside. Mix 1 CUP flour, salt & pepper, smoked paprika, and 2 rosemary sprigs finely chopped in Ziploc baggie and set aside.

Rinse chicken in cold water, pat dry and add salt & pepper both sides. Place chicken in baggie with flour mixture and shake bag to lightly coat.

Over medium to high heat place large skillet and add canola oil. When oil is hot, add chicken and cook until golden brown on all sides, but not fully cooked, then remove to plate. Coat the bottom of a roasting pan with olive oil and add chicken and vegetables, chopped sage leaves and remaining rosemary sprigs, pour a little olive oil over vegetables, just enough to coat them and a pinch of salt and pepper (optional). Cover and bake for 1 hour, test for doneness. Chicken fluids should run clear & veggies should be tender.

When chicken is done remove to serving platter, place vegetable around chicken, garnish with cooked rosemary sprigs and cover with foil.

Place roasting pan on stove top over medium heat, whisk in 3 tablespoons of flour until well blended, about 2-3 minutes, add chicken broth to desired consistency, pour gravy over chicken and vegetables and serve.

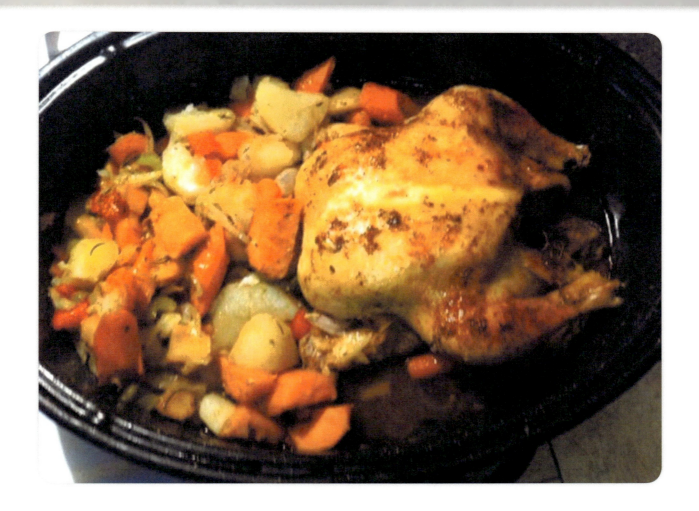

**NOTE:** Store uncooked chicken backs and wing tips in freezer to use for chicken broth – good in freezer for up to 3 - 6 months. For Chicken Broth; place chicken parts in large pot and cover with cold water. Add onion, celery, carrots, bay leaf, salt & pepper and let simmer for about 1 hour. Place in Mason Jar (leaving 1" of space at the top of the jar) and place in freezer for up to 6 months. Or you can use an airtight plastic container or a Ziploc Freezer bag.

# Baked Chicken Stew with Herbed Goat Cheese Mashed Potatoes

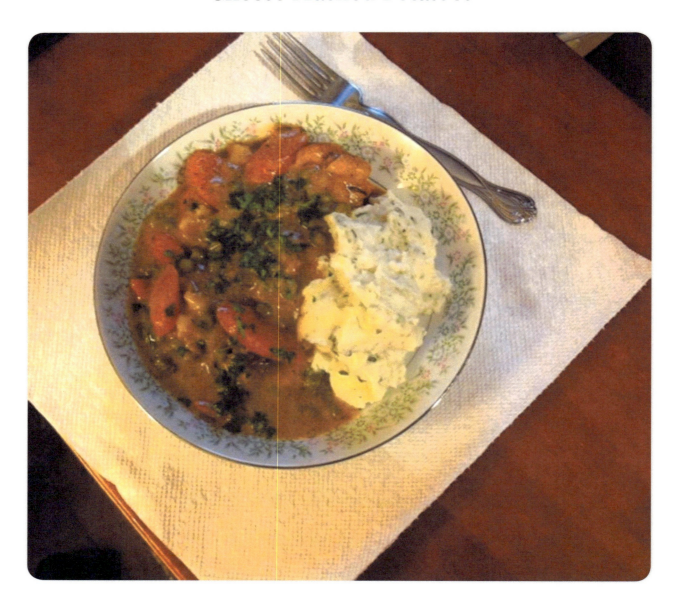

# Baked Chicken Stew

**INGREDIENTS**:

1 Whole Organic Chicken – cut up

3 Cups sliced carrots – ½" diagonal (about 4 medium size carrots

1 Cup of frozen baby peas

2 Celery Stalks sliced ½" slices

1 Large Sweet Onion sliced

4 Garlic Cloves minced

4 Tablespoons freshly chopped Rosemary

4 Tablespoons All-Purpose Flour

3 Cups Chicken Broth (or so)

½ Cup of Half and Half

All-Purpose Seasoning

Salt & Pepper to taste

2 Tablespoons of Extra Virgin Olive Oil

2 Tablespoons of unsalted butter

**DIRECTIONS**:

Brine Chicken the night before.

THE NEXT DAY:

PREHEAT OVEN TO 350⁰

Rinse chicken well and pat dry with paper towels. Season with All-Purpose Season, cover the meat well and let sit for 15 minutes.

Heat olive oil and melt butter in a frying pan. When oil and butter are hot, add chicken and brown on each side place chicken in an oven-proof dish with a cover. In same pan add garlic and Rosemary stir well lifting flavors from the bottom of the pan. Sauté for about 3-5 minutes; stir in flour mix well and gradually add chicken stock to desired thickness; mix well and whisk in Half & Half, continue until broth is a nice thick consistency.

Pour carrots, onion and peas over chicken then pour in the broth. Add salt & pepper to taste. Bake at 350⁰ for 2 hours stirring occasionally. When chicken is falling off the bones, it is ready.

Serve with Baked Mashed Potatoes with Herb and Garlic Goat Cheese and a nice crusty French bread.

# Turmeric and Lemon Roasted Chicken with Vegetables

**INGREDIENTS**:

2.5 LB Whole Chicken

1 stick of unsalted butter – softened

6 sprigs of fresh thyme leaves

2 sprigs of fresh rosemary leaves chopped

2 quarter wedges of preserved lemon – rinsed and pulp removed and chopped

2 garlic cloves – minced

Kosher Salt

Coarse pepper

Turmeric

Paprika

2 tablespoons of All Purpose Poultry Seasoning – recipe on page 16

3 carrots – peeled and sliced in ½' slices on the diagonal

4 medium sized red potatoes slice in ½ slices

1 onion chopped

½ cup of fresh chopped parsley

3 tablespoon of all-purpose flour

Extra Virgin Olive Oil

**DIRECTIONS**:

Brine Chicken the night before; the next day remove chicken from brine and rinse very well inside and outside in cold water. Pat dry with paper towels and set aside.

In a small bowl add softened butter, 1 teaspoon of Kosher salt, 2 teaspoons of turmeric,1 tablespoon of pepper, 3 sprigs of thyme leaves and 1 sprig of chopped rosemary leaves, lemon, garlic, 1 tablespoon of All Purpose Poultry seasonings – mix well and place in refrigerator.

Cut your vegetables and place in a Ziplock bag and add 1 teaspoon of salt, 2 tablespoons black pepper, ½ teaspoon of turmeric, chopped parsley and ¼ cup of olive – shake well to coat vegetables.

Carefully lift the skin away for the meat of the chicken with your fingers. With a spoon place butter mixture under the skin of chicken, front, back and legs, and a spoonful in the cavity along with salt and pepper 1 sprig of rosemary and 3 sprigs thyme. Sprinkle the chicken with 2 teaspoons of salt, 1 tablespoon of pepper, 1 tablespoon of turmeric.

In large roasting pan pour enough olive oil in pan to coat the bottom. Place the chicken in the pan toward the top leaving space at the bottom to add your vegetables.

Cook covered for 1 hour at 350 degrees for 1 hour or 15 minutes per pound. Remove cover, check for doneness (temperature should be should 165 degrees – insert meat thermometer into the inner thigh, near the bone but not touching it.

# Nina and Darrell's Sweet Wine and Chicken Medallions

## INGREDIENTS:

4 boneless chicken breast – cut in 1" medallions

8 baby portabella mushrooms – sliced

1 cup chopped fresh parsley

10 strips of bacon – sliced thin

4 tablespoons olive oil

1.5 sticks unsalted butter - divided

1.5 cups of sweet white wine

½ cup chicken stock

1 cup and ¼ cup all-purpose flour - divided

3 Whole garlic cloves – paper removed

All Purpose Season

## DIRECTIONS:

The day before cut chicken in inch medallions sprinkle with all purpose season. Place in plastic bag and place on the bottom shelf in the refrigerator.

The next day remove chicken from refrigerator an hour before preparation.

Heat skillet and add olive oil. When oil is hot add garlic cloves to infuse the oil – let garlic saute garlic until brown, do not let it burn. Remove from and discard.

In a Ziplock bag add 1 cup flour and ½ cup of all purpose season. Coat chicken with flour, shake off excess and place on a paper towel.

In a large black skillet on high heat add ½ stick of butter and 4 tablespoons of olive oil and 2 garlic cloves to infuse the oil, remove cloves before they burn. When oil is hot add chicken and brown on each side – until golden brown. Remove chicken from skillet and set aside. In the same skillet add bacon and mushrooms and cook until mushrooms are brown and bacon is done. Add ¼ cup flour stirring for about 2 minutes, add wine and chicken stock and continue to cook and stir for 2 more minutes or until sauce starts to thicken. Then add ¼ cup of all purpose season and stir well. Add chicken and let simmer for 10 minutes or until chicken is done – garnish with parsley and serve.

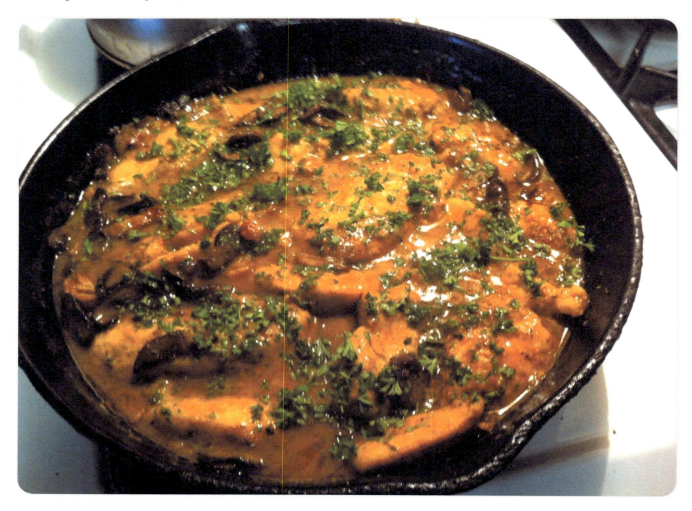

# My Classic Fried Chicken

Buttermilk, lots of garlic, some rosemary, fresh sage leaves, and some dried thyme make this chicken not just moist, but full of flavor. My friend Vicky is not much of a chicken eater, but she loves my fried chicken. This method may take some time, but it is worth it and even best if left to marinade overnight. Use your favorite chicken parts or have your butcher cut up a whole chicken. For this recipe I am going to use chicken parts. For best results us a cast iron skillet.

Serves 6 - 8

**INGREDIENTS**:

| | |
|---|---|
| 6 wings – tips removed | 6 thighs |
| 6 legs | 2 large breasts (cut in half) |

**THE BRINE**

| | |
|---|---|
| Kosher salt | 6 sprigs of fresh rosemary |
| Freshly ground black pepper | 10 sage leaves |
| 1 quart cultured buttermilk | 5 tablespoons of dried thyme |
| 1 garlic small garlic bulb | |

Rinse chicken parts under cold water, pat dry with paper towels and place in large plastic bowl. Salt & pepper both sides thoroughly then cover with buttermilk, add whole garlic cloves, rosemary, sage and thyme, cover and refrigerate overnight or at least 4 hours.

### Let's Fry Some Chicken

In large plastic Ziplock bag add:

| | |
|---|---|
| 3 cups of flour | 4 tables of course black pepper |
| 4 tablespoons of smoked paprika | 4 tablespoons of onion powder |
| 3 tablespoons of kosher salt | 4 tablespoons of garlic powder |

Shake bag to mix seasonings well with the flour

48 oz. Pure Vegetable Oil
Large black skillet
Flame medium to high heat

If using a black skillet frying pan, to test your oil for readiness, add a pinch of flour to the hot oil, if it bubbles and fries, it is ready!

## *Pan-Fried Chicken*

The two main keys to making perfect fried chicken are the temperature of the oil and the actual steps of frying.

Choose oils with a high smoke point: vegetable shortening or oil, peanut oil or canola oil are all good choices.

- To get truly golden-brown and crispy chicken, use a cast iron skillet. You can't beat cast iron for even heat distribution and reliable frying.

- The fat should be about one inch deep in the skillet, coming about halfway up the food.

- Get the oil good and hot before adding the chicken: about 350 degrees F (175 degrees C).

- Using tongs, carefully lower chicken pieces into the oil skin-side down.

- Fry in batches: overcrowding the pan will lower the temperature of the oil, causing the chicken to be soggy and greasy.

- When the chicken pieces are a deep golden brown, remove them to a cooling rack set over a baking sheet to catch any drips. Insert an instant-read thermometer into the chicken to make sure it is fully cooked before moving on to the next batch. The USDA recommends the internal temperature should be around 165 degrees F; however I prefer my chicken be about 180 degrees F.

Good old fashioned mashed potatoes and your favorite green veg compliments this chicken perfectly!!

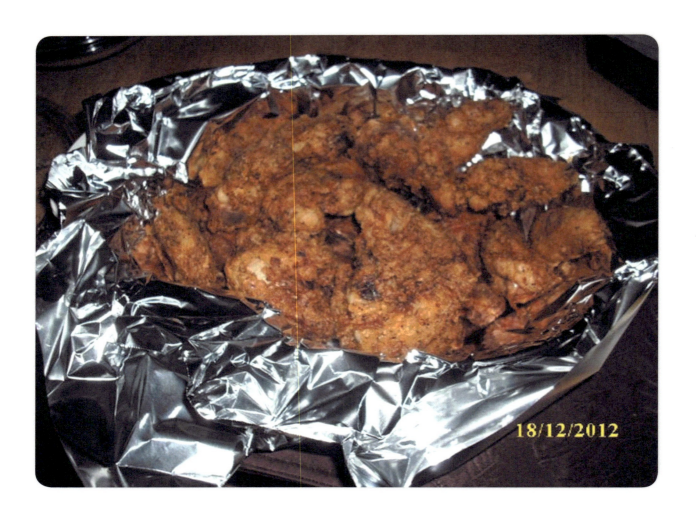

18/12/2012

# BEEF AND PORK

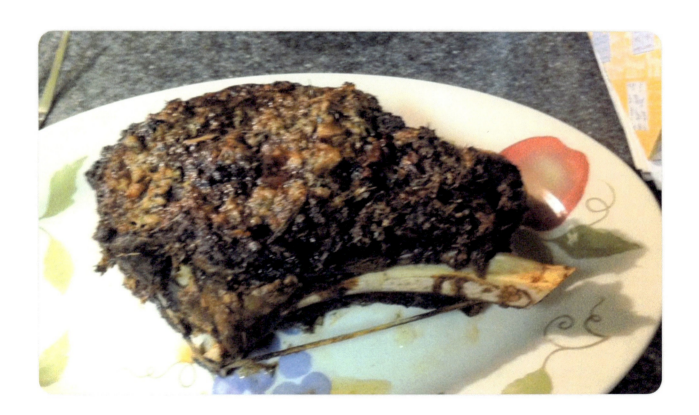

# Baby Back Ribs with Honey-Ginger Barbeque Sauce

You can double or triple the dry rub and keep it in a Mason jar or whatever airtight jar or Ziploc bag you have. It will keep for up to 6 months the same goes for the sauce which freezes well.

## INGREDIENTS:

1 Rack of Lean Baby Back Ribs – rinsed and patted dry

## DRY RUB FOR RIBS:

2 teaspoon kosher salt

2 teaspoons of freshly ground black pepper

2 tablespoons smoked paprika

1 tablespoon onion powder

2 tablespoons garlic powder

2 tablespoons dark brown sugar

Place ingredients in a small bowl and blend well. Rub seasons on both sides of ribs then wrap the ribs tightly in cellophane, place on plate and put on the bottom shelf of refrigerate and let sit at least 8 hours or overnight.

## THE SAUCE:

Chop your veggies and have them ready!

2 tablespoons unsalted butter

4 lemons – zest of one, 2 sliced & 2 juiced

2 tablespoons freshly chopped parsley

2 tablespoons freshly chopped basil leaves – about 8 leaves

½ cup extra virgin olive oil & 1 tablespoon

½ cup ketchup

1 cup honey

4 garlic cloves – finely chopped

1 large Vidalia onion – diced

¼ cup apple cider vinegar

1 knob of ginger (about 1 inch) skinned and grated

½ teaspoon kosher salt

1 teaspoon coarse black pepper

In medium sauce pan heat 2 tablespoon of butter, onion, garlic, and ginger and sauté for about 3 minutes until fragrant; add lemon slices & juice, ketchup, olive oil and vinegar, bring to a boil then reduce heat and simmer for 1 hour stirring occasionally. Add honey and herbs and let simmer for 30 minutes continue to stir occasional to be sure ingredients are blended well. Place in food processor or use immersion blender.

## PREHEAT OVEN TO 350⁰

Cover bottom of roasting pan with barbeque sauce, add ribs and pour more sauce on top of ribs. Cover pan and cook for 1 hour or until tender. I like them to fall off the bone!

# Baked Pork Chops with Apples

Apples and Pork are a delicious combination; the savory flavor of the pork and the bitter-sweet tang of the Granny Smith Apples, makes this a very hearty dish.

## INGREDIENTS:

6 center cut pork chops

4 Granny Smith Apples-peeled and thinly sliced

2 small bunch of scallions –thinly sliced

3 tablespoons of unsalted butter

3 tablespoon of extra virgin olive oil – divided

4 garlic cloves – minced

1 tablespoon fresh rosemary – finely chopped

¼ cup freshly chopped parsley (about ½ bunch)

## RUB FOR PORK CHOPS:

5 tables of finely chopped – fresh rosemary – (about 4-5 sprigs)

5 tablespoons ground sage

2 tablespoons of cinnamon

½ teaspoon of ground nutmeg

¾ cup of light brown sugar

2 teaspoon of kosher salt

2 tablespoons course black pepper

Mix well

This should be enough to rub your meat and to sprinkle over apples.

Preheat oven 350⁰

Rinse the pork chops under cool water, pat dry and apply your Pork Rub on both sides, then set them aside or rub the night before, wrap in cellophane, place in refrigerator on bottom shelf until ready to use. The longer they marinade the more intense the flavor. Remove from refrigerator at least 30 minutes before placing in oven.

In skillet melt butter, add 2 tablespoons of olive oil, when hot add chops and brown on each side, about 2 minutes each side. Remove from heat and set aside.

Cover the bottom of a 9x13 baking dish with 1 tablespoon of olive oil. Layer sliced apples on the bottom, sprinkle apples with the remaining pork rub. Layer pork chops on top of apples, and add minced garlic, chopped rosemary and sliced scallions over chops.

Cover dish with foil and bake 35 minutes, remove foil and bake another 20 minutes, until chops are done and tender. Sprinkle with fresh parsley and serve with a green vegetable.

# Beef and Broccoli Stir Fry

Chinese Food is one of my favorite types of cuisine. The recipes always require the freshest ingredients. Actually, Chinese Food is one of the few things I miss since my move to North Carolina from Boston 10 years ago. Every trip I make up north; be it Boston or visiting relatives in New York or New Jersey, one of our first stops is to the Chinese restaurant. But I have found I can fulfill my craving for "good" Chinese food by making my own and giving it any twist that I like.

## INGREDIENTS:

1 egg

7 tablespoons of soy sauce – divided

2 tablespoons of dark brown sugar - divided

2 knobs of fresh ginger – divided – 1 piece coarsely chopped; the other piece grated

4 garlic cloves – divided – 2 cloves cut in pieces; the other grated

1 lb. top round steak, thinly sliced in bite size pieces

2 bunches fresh baby broccoli or broccolini flowerets, stems removed*

4 tbsp. peanut oil

6 green onions, sliced

½ cup of water

2 tbsp. cornstarch

½ cup chopped chives – cut with scissors

## MARINADE FOR BEEF

In bowl, mix together, egg, 3 tablespoons of soy sauce, 1 tablespoon brown sugar, 1 knob of coarsely chopped ginger and 2 cloves of garlic cut in pieces, mix well, add steak and set in refrigerator for at least 4 hours or overnight. Discard marinade when done.

## DIRECTIONS:

In hot wok or hot skillet add 2 tablespoons of oil. Add beef and sauté until tender (about 5-8 minutes); remove beef and set aside. Add remaining 2 tablespoons oil and sauté broccoli, grated ginger, grated garlic and green onions for 5 minutes. In a small bowl mix water, soy sauce, cornstarch, and sugar; pour mixture over vegetables, stir until combined. Add meat and cover. Reduce heat and simmer until broccoli is tender (5-10 minutes) and sauce has thickened. Serve over rice. Serves 3 - 6.

Garnish with chives.

*Place broccoli stems in plastic bag reserve for broccoli soup by placing them in the freezer. They will keep for 3 months.

# GRILLED POT ROAST With A TANGY SAUCE

One of my favorite markets to do my grocery shopping often has a buy one get one sale on London Broil, however, when I returned home to prepare my London Broil for the grill, I discovered I had purchased a 5lb pot roast in error, so I grilled it and it was delicious. I prepared it the same way I had planned for the London broil. Basting meat frequently with a tangy sauce.

## INGREDIENTS:

1 – 2-3LB Pot Roast

## THE MARINADE:

Mix together:

2 teaspoons of kosher salt

2 teaspoons of black coarse pepper

2 tablespoons of onion powder

6 crushed garlic cloves

3 tablespoons of Worcestershire Sauce

½ cup red wine vinegar

4 tablespoons of extra virgin olive oil

Juice of 1 lemon

2 tablespoons chopped rosemary leaves

Poke holes in the meat with a fork and place in a Ziploc bag and pour marinade on top. Seal bag and keep in refrigerator overnight or at least 8 hours. Discard marinade when done.

Prepare your grill and place meat on direct heat to sear, about 3 -5 minutes each side. Then place on indirect heat and cook to your liking. Baste with sauce frequently.

Use your meat thermometer to gauge to your preference.

## THE TANGY SAUCE:
## INGREDIENTS:

2 sweet onions – diced

1 red bell pepper – diced

1 jalapeno pepper – seed, ribbed and diced

1 quart of your canned (seeded) tomatoes or 2 cans crushed tomatoes

1 small knob of fresh ginger – grated – about 1 tablespoon

4 garlic cloves – minced

2 cups chicken stock

(Tangy Sauce con't)

1 tablespoon Worcestershire Sauce

1 tablespoon red wine vinegar

1 tablespoon molasses

1 lemon – zest & juice

1 orange – zest & juice

1 cup ketchup

1 teaspoon ground cinnamon

1 tablespoon chili powder

¼ cup brown sugar

## DIRECTIONS:

In medium size stock pot heat olive oil add, garlic, onions, jalapeno and bell pepper, sauté until soft, stir in ginger, tomatoes, chicken broth, Worcestershire sauce, vinegar, molasses, lemon & orange zest & juice, ketchup, cinnamon, chili powder & sugar, bring to a boil. Then reduce heat and let simmer for

about 1 hour until it thickens.

Place sauce in blender and liquefy or use an immersion blender.

# Savory Beef Stew

## INGREDIENTS:

1.5 LBS of stew beef (Chuck Roast cut in cubes)

All Purpose Seasoning (see recipe below)

2 tablespoons unsalted butter

2 tablespoons extra virgin olive oil

1 large onion diced

6 garlic cloves minced

6 medium russet potatoes – (about 5 cups) cut in
   bite size cubes

4 carrots cut in ½" slices on the diagonal

1 cup sliced portabella mushrooms

½ cup red wine

1 teaspoon liquid smoke

4 ounces tomato paste

1 tablespoon white granulated sugar

2 tablespoons Worcestershire Sauce

2 tablespoon ketchup

32 ounces of beef broth

1 quart canned tomatoes (or 1/28 oz. can of whole
   tomatoes)

1 teaspoon dried thyme

2 tablespoons all-purpose flour

Salt & Pepper to taste

4 tablespoons of freshly chopped parsley

## ALL PURPOSE SEASONING:

¼ cup each: Kosher Salt, Coarse Black Pepper, Smoke Paprika, Onion Powder, Garlic Powder

2 tablespoons dried thyme (store remaining seasoning in air tight container or a Mason Jar)

## DIRECTIONS:

Dry beef with a paper towel, place in bowl and coat with All Purpose Seasoning (about 3 tablespoons). In large pot heat olive and butter; when butter has melted add some of the beef, one layer (you will do this in two batches). Brown then remove to plate and brown the remaining and set aside. In same pot add the garlic and onions, wine and stir well. Add the broth, bring to a boil and add the beef along with the juices. Let simmer for two hours. Mix 2 tablespoons of flour with 1 cup of the broth from the stew and mix well; add to pot; then add the potatoes, carrot and tomatoes, give a good stir and cook until potatoes and carrots are tender. Taste and add salt & pepper if necessary. Stir in the parsley and serve.

# Ham and Potatoes Sautéed with Rosemary

"Waste not – want not," could possibly be one of my favorite mottos because I do not like to waste food and I very seldom throw food away. I also have a Chocolate Lab, Harmoney, so if we don't eat it, he will. Well this recipe was created after we purchased a very large Smithfield ham at a very good price. I baked it, cut it in half, ate off of half for Sunday and Monday dinner, had ham slices for sandwiches and ham salad as a fabulous addition to a garden salad; the other half went to the freezer which will keep very well for up to 3 month just be sure to wrap it tightly in cellophane and aluminum foil. When ready remove it from the freezer and let it thaw in the bottom of the refrigerator for about 2 days.

## INGREDIENTS:

1 tablespoons of Extra Virgin Olive Oil

4 tablespoons unsalted butter

2 large leeks – sliced and washed* well

1 small Spanish onion – diced

8-10 small red potatoes – skin removed on and
    diced

2 teaspoons of kosher salt

2 teaspoons of black ground pepper

4 garlic cloves minced

1-2 sprig of fresh rosemary – about 2 tablespoons

5 cups of diced cooked ham

## DIRECTIONS:

In large sauce pan add olive oil, butter, when butter has melted add the Rosemary and potatoes, salt and pepper, stir it up well then cover pan and cook for 10 - 15 minutes, stirring occasionally. Add leeks and garlic Remove lid and continue to cook for another 10 minutes, turning flame a bit higher to give potatoes a nice crispy texture, cook until potatoes are soft, but firm. Taste for seasoned satisfaction. Add ham and heat through. When ham is hot, remove from heat and serve.

*Cleaning Leeks: Leeks are root vegetables they are a member of the onion family, but with a much milder flavor. To thoroughly clean them, fill a bowl with cool, clean water and add your sliced Leeks and swish around a bit with your fingers and all of the dirt particles will fall to the bottom of the bowl.

# Herb Crusted Pork Rib Roast

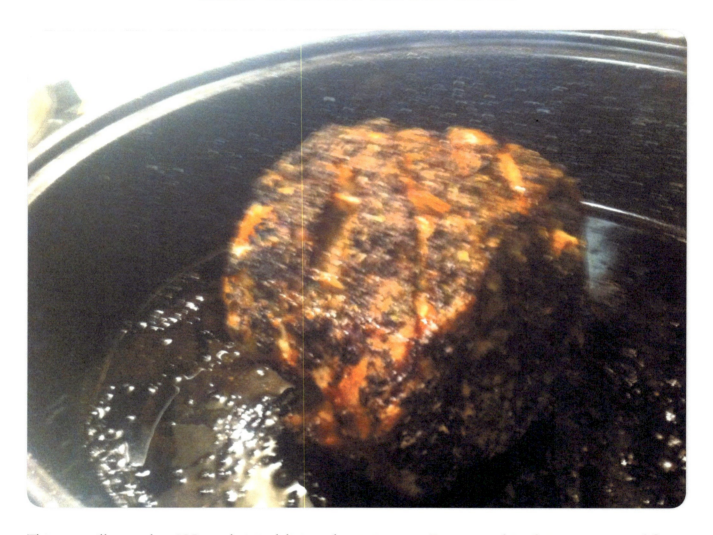

This one will wow them! Not only is it delicious, but it is pretty. For me, nothing brings out natural flavor of a good piece of meat like fresh garden herbs. The sauce requires a broth, go for the vegetable – homemade vegetable broth with shallots, mild & sweet.

# Herb Crusted Rib Roast

**INGREDIENTS:**

THE "STAR!" 2.5 lb. pork rib roast

**THE NIGHT BEFORE**:

Wet Rub: 4 tablespoons each of finely chopped fresh herbs: Rosemary, Sage, Thyme, 1 teaspoon kosher salt, 2 teaspoons grated fresh garlic, 1 tablespoon ground black pepper, 2 -3 tablespoons of extra virgin olive oil, mixed well.

Score fat side of roast, rub herbs on roast, wrap in cellophane and let sit over night or at least 4 hours.

**THE NEXT DAY OR 4 HOURS LATER:**

Preheat oven to 500⁰ - set pork rib roast in shallow roasting pan, fat side up – roast for 45 minutes to sear the meat. Then reduce your oven to 325⁰ and 20 minutes per pound. 2.5 lb. roast - 2 hour and 30 minutes - meat thermometer should read 145 - remove to platter, cover with foil and let sit for 20 minutes before serving.

**THE SAUCE:**

3 shallots finely chopped

3 tablespoons of unsalted butter

3 cloves grated fresh garlic

3 teaspoons of chopped rosemary

1 teaspoon of finely chopped sage

1 teaspoon of fresh thyme leaves – about 5 sprigs

3 tablespoons of flour

1/2 cup to 1 cup of good white wine (depending on your preference of consistency and taste)

1/2 cup of half and half

3 tablespoons of chicken or vegetable broth

Salt and pepper to taste (start with ½ teaspoon each)

In saucepan melt butter, add shallots and cook until they wilt (about 5 mins.), add garlic and herbs, cook for another 2 minutes. Add flour and make your roux....cook for at least a minute to cook off the flour taste. Add wine, broth, 1/2 & ½, broth, salt & pepper to taste, bring to boil, and then simmer until it thickens. Taste to meet your expectations and add what your taste buds desire. Set aside and serve with you perfect pork

I serve this with roasted red potatoes, asparagus and herbed biscuits (same herbs used in the roast). I like to keep the same flavors and herbs throughout my meal.

# Herbed 3-Meat Meat Loaf with Mushroom Gravy

I was never big fan of meat loaf growing up. I always felt it was "missing" something, more flavor. Here is my version of a "tasty" meatloaf. It seems like a big effort for meat loaf, but for me, it is worth it. Make it for Sunday Dinner! Add some Buttered-Smashed Yukon Potatoes & Apple, and roasted Asparagus and herb biscuits and maybe a Chocolate Mousse for dessert.

## INGREDIENTS:

1 stick & 3 tablespoon unsalted butter - divided

1 large sweet onion – diced

4 garlic cloves – minced

1 medium red pepper – diced

1 medium yellow pepper – diced

1 pint sliced Portobello mushrooms sliced - divided

½ lb. chopped sirloin

¼ lb. ground pork

¼ ground white turkey

1 cup of buttered panko bread crumbs (recipe below)

1 large egg – beaten

1 teaspoon of kosher salt

1 tablespoon of Worcestershire sauce

4 oz. jar (1/2 cup) drained whole tomatoes (reserve the juice) chopped

2 tablespoons light brown sugar

2 tablespoon ground black pepper

2 slices toasted rye bread - crumbled

2 tablespoons sour cream

8 fresh sage leaves – finely chopped

2 tablespoons finely chopped marjoram leaves or 1 tablespoon dried

6 sprigs of thyme – leaves removed – chopped

¼ cup fresh parsley – chopped

3 tablespoons of all-purpose flour

½ cup of red wine

## DIRECTIONS: Preheat over 350⁰

## BUTTERED BREAD CRUMBS RECIPE:

Melt 6 tablespoons butter in medium size sauté pan on medium heat, add bread crumbs and sauté until butter has been absorbed into the breadcrumbs and breadcrumbs are golden brown. Remove from heat and set aside. Meatloaf: In large saucepan melt 2 tablespoons of butter over medium heat; add onions, garlic, peppers, and 1 cup of mushrooms. Sauté vegetables until soft, remove from heat, set aside and let cool.

In large bowl add meat, bread crumbs, egg, salt, Worcestershire sauce, tomatoes, brown sugar, pepper, bread, sour cream, herbs and cooked vegetables. Using your hands mix all the ingredients together until well combined, but do not over mix. Shape meat into a loaf and bake covered for 40 minutes, remove cover check and cook for an addition 15 – 20 minutes. Meatloaf is done when internal temperature reaches 160⁰. Remove from pan and cover with foil, let rest for 10 minutes. Reserve pan juices.

## MUSHROOM GRAVY:

In medium sauce melt 3 tablespoon of unsalted butter, add remaining mushrooms and sauté about 3-5 minutes until soft. Add flour and mix for at 2 minutes, add 2 tablespoons of pan juices (as close as you can come to 2 tablespoons, depending on what juices are in pan). Add wine – taste and add salt and/or pepper if necessary. Stir over medium-low flame until gravy thickens.

My mom loves Italian sausage and she loves rice, maybe not as much as she love potatoes, but we will get to that later. Brown rice was not, notice I said was not her favorite, but this recipe changed her mind. If you are not a fan of brown rice, your mind will be changed too. This recipe is savory and earthy and the flavor of the Italian sausage combined with the peppers and onions rocks! Check it out!

# Italian Sausage with Brown Rice

### Serves 3 -6

## INGREDIENTS:

1 lb. of Sweet Italian Beef Sausage

2 cups of brown whole grain rice*

3 tablespoons of extra virgin olive oil

2 tablespoons of freshly chopped parsley

2 tablespoons of freshly chopped oregano

1 onion sliced

½ red bell pepper diced

½ green bell pepper diced

1 garlic clove finely chopped

## DIRECTIONS:

Cook rice according to instructions. Drain, let cool and place in refrigerator for at least 1 hour.

Preheat oven to 350°

In small pan add 1 tablespoon of olive oil and Italian sausage. Bake for 30 minutes, let cool then slice in ½ inch slices and set aside

In large sauté pan 2 tablespoons of olive oil, onions, peppers, and garlic. Cook until vegetables are soft, about 5-8 minutes. Add rice and let heat through, about 5 minutes. Then add sausage, sprinkle herbs on top, cover, reduce heat and let simmer about 10 minutes then serve.

*Saffron rice is a great alternative.

RECIPE: Melt 2 tablespoons of unsalted butter in medium sauce pan, stir in 1 cup of rice stir in butter until coated. Add 2 cups of water and about 8 saffron threads. Bring to boil, lower heat, cover and simmer about 10 minutes, or until light and fluffy. Remove from heat and let cool and place in refrigerator for about 3 hours. Refrigerating the rice keeps the grains separate when adding to your cooked ingredients.

# POTATOES, RICE AND VEGETABLES

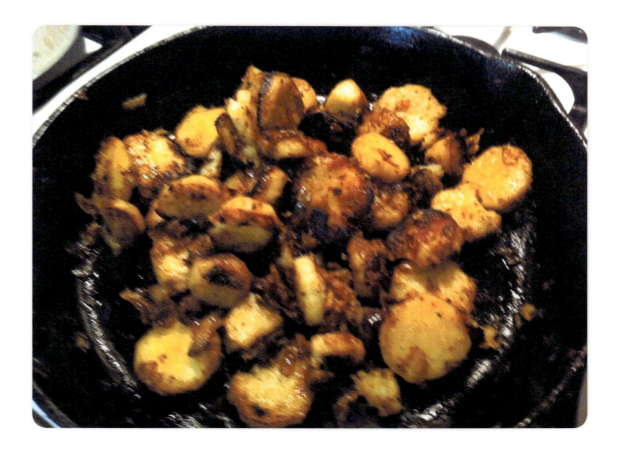

**Sautéd White Sweet Potatoes**

*Recipe on page page 81*

# Butter Rice with Veggies

## INGREDIENTS:

1 cup of brown rice – cooked per directions

1 stick of unsalted butter

1 carrot sliced

1 cup of edamame – steamed

1 Vidalia onion sliced

1 garlic clove – minced

½ cup of sliced portabella mushrooms

1 cup of freshly chopped parsley

Salt & Pepper to taste

*Use left over rice or cook the rice and place in the refrigerator until cold.*

In large sauté pan add ½ stick of butter and carrots. Sauté carrots for about 5 minutes, then add the garlic, onion and mushrooms, sauté until onions and mushrooms have wilted, stirring occasionally. Add the edamame and sauté for about 5 minutes. Add the rice and as much of the left over butter that is to your liking (generally end up using the whole stick). Stir and salt & pepper to taste. Add the parsley and serve.

NOTE: You can add cooked shrimp or cooked chicken to make this a one pan meal.

# Sautéd White Sweet Potatoes

## INGREDIENTS:

3 medium sized white sweet potatoes – peeled and cut in ½ slices

2 tablespoon extra-virgin coconut oil

3 caramelized onions (see recipe below)

Salt

½ packed light brown sugar

2 teaspoons of nutmeg

1 tablespoon cinnamon

## DIRECTIONS:

**Caramelized Onions**: Slice 3 or 4 large onions and place them in a skillet with 2 tablespoons of olive oil (add more if needed). Let the onions sauté, stirring occasionally, until they become a nice dark brown, but not burnt.

**NOTE***: Cook a batch and keep them in the refrigerator. They are great on burgers, hot dogs, sandwiches or to enhance any vegetable. They will keep in the refrigerator for about 4 weeks.*

In a heavy skillet, I used a good old cast iron on medium heat add the coconut oil, it melts quickly. Add potatoes, stir to coat with the oil. Add nutmeg, cinnamon, ½ teaspoon of Kosher salt and stir well.
Cover and let steam for about 15 minutes. Remove cover, and cook until browned and done, about 20 minutes. Add onions and cook for another 5 minutes. You want them to be a bit charded and crispy on the outside and soft and sweet on the inside.

# Roasted Broccoli and Cauliflower

**INGREDIENTS:**

1 medium cauliflower – cut up into flowerets

1 medium broccoli – cup up into flowerets

2 - 4 tablespoons of extra virgin olive oil

4 garlic cloves, minced

1 teaspoon salt

1 tablespoon ground pepper

Parmesan Cheese – freshly grated

**DIRECTIONS:**

Place vegetables on a baking sheet and drizzle with olive oil. Mix well to cover vegetables with oil. Add salt & pepper and bake at 450° for 25 minutes or until slightly browned. Sprinkle with freshly grated Parmesan cheese and serve.

# Garlic Smashed Potato Bake

## **INGREDIENTS:**

5 pounds russet, peeled and cut in cubes

6 chopped garlic cloves

4 cups of vegetable broth – enough to just cover potatoes

1 cup of half and half to start may need to add for consistency

4 green onions, chopped

¼ cup of fresh chopped parsley leaves

¼ cup of fresh chopped cilantro leaves

1 teaspoon salt

1 teaspoon garlic powder (optional)

1 stick unsalted butter – divided

4 ounces of whipped cream cheese

## **DIRECTIONS:**

Preheat the oven to 375 degrees. Butter casserole dish and set aside.

Place the potatoes and garlic in a large pot and cover with broth and salt; boil the potatoes until tender.

Drain potatoes and garlic and return them to the pot. Mash the potatoes and garlic add 6 tablespoons of butter (slice so it will melt easier), half and half gradually to preference, cream cheese, onions, pepper, cilantro and parsley. Use hand blender and mix well to desired consistency. Scoop the potatoes into the prepared baking pan. Dot potatoes with 2 tablespoons butter. Bake for 20-25 minutes until the potatoes are lightly browned on top and heated through.

# Mashed Potatoes with Parsley & Cilantro

Potatoes are like poultry, there are so many things you can do with them. This potato recipe went great with the Basil Baked Pork Chops.

## INGREDIENTS:

4 Cups of diced All Purpose Potatoes

2 cups of chicken or vegetable broth

4 garlic cloves, minced

½ cup half & half

¼ cup finely chopped parsley

¼ cup finely chopped cilantro

2 tablespoon of Basil Pesto

6 tablespoons of butter

½ teaspoon of kosher salt (to taste)

1 teaspoon of white pepper (to taste)

Parsley & Cilantro for garnish

## DIRECTIONS:

In large pot add vegetable broth and potatoes. Bring to a boil, lower heat and simmer for about 20 minutes, until potatoes are tender. Drain potatoes, but save the broth. In large bowl add potatoes, butter, garlic, parsley, cilantro and basil, salt & pepper then mash. Using a hand mixer, blend in the half and half and 2 tablespoons of the reserved vegetable broth – optional. Taste, garnish and serve.

# Mashed Yukon's & Granny Smith's Apples

## INGREDIENTS:

3 lbs Baby Yukon Gold Potatoes – peeled and cut in half

3 Granny Smith Apples – peeled and grated

6 garlic cloves minced

2 cups of half and half

4 tablespoons of unsalted butter

1 teaspoon kosher salt

1 teaspoon white pepper

## DIRECTIONS:

In large pot add potatoes, apples, garlic and half and half (enough to cover the potatoes), salt & pepper. Bring to boil lower heat and simmer until potatoes are soft, about 20 minutes. Remove from heat, either drain and reserve excess half and half or ad more, depending on the consistency that you prefer. Add the butter and mix using a hand mixer until potatoes are nice and smooth. Taste for salt content and serve.

# Oven Roasted Baby Red Potatoes

## INGREDIENTS:

3 lbs (one small bag) baby red potatoes

4 minced garlic cloves (use garlic press)

1 stick of unsalted butter - melted

1 teaspoon sea salt

1 ½ teaspoons ground black pepper

1 cup fresh chopped parsley

## DIRECTIONS:

Preheat oven to 375°

Butter a large roasting pan or casserole dish and set aside. Depending on the size of the potatoes cut them in half or quarters. Place potatoes in dish add garlic, butter, salt, pepper and mix it up. Place uncover in oven and bake for 15 minutes, remove from oven add parsley, cover and bake for 45 minutes, until done, stirring often to be sure flavors coat all the potatoes evenly. When done you can place under broiler for a few minutes if you want them browned more. Add some more fresh parsley just before serving.

# Kale, Potato & Pancetta

**INGREDIENTS:**

8 cups of fresh kale – roughly chopped – not
   packed

4 Medium size all-purpose potatoes – diced

1 oz. diced pancetta

3 garlic cloves – minced

½ teaspoon of salt

1 teaspoon of coarse black pepper

1 tablespoons of unsalted butter

¼ chopped fresh parsley

**DIRECTIONS:**

In medium pot ad potatoes and cover with water, bring to a boil, lower heat and simmer until potatoes are done out 15 minutes; drain and set aside.

In large sauce pan add pancetta and cook until crisp, remove pancetta with slotted spoon and set aside. In same sauce pan add kale and sauté until wilted, salt and pepper, butter, potatoes, pancetta and parsley.

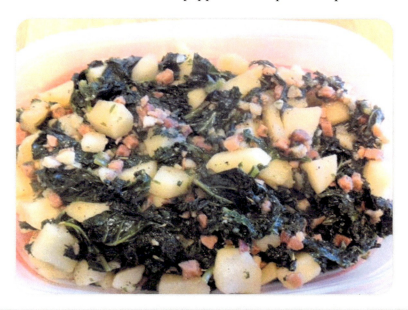

# Roasted Rosemary & Thyme Potatoes

**<u>INGREDIENTS</u>:**

6 Medium Russet Potatoes cut in wedges

2 tables of extra virgin olive oil

2 small sprigs of fresh rosemary chopped (2
  tablespoons dried)

2 teaspoons dried thyme

1 tablespoon kosher salt

1 tablespoon coarse black pepper

2 tablespoon melted unsalted butter (optional)

Ziploc bag – place prepared vegetables, herbs, slat
  & pepper in bag and shake to coat.

Preheat Oven to 400˚

On cookie sheet place vegetables in a single layer. Roast for 20 – 30 minutes. Check for tenderness, with a fork or toothpick. Serve as is or pour melted butter over potatoes and place under broiler until nice and browned.

# Green Bean and Tomatoes With Fresh Basil

**INGREDIENTS:**

2 lbs. fresh green beans – ends snipped – left whole

1 ½ cups of vegetable broth – enough to just cover
 the beans

½ stick of unsalted butter

3 garlic cloves – minced

¼ cup of brown - packed

1 tablespoon of black pepper

½ teaspoon of kosher salt

3 cups grape or cherry tomatoes – cut in half

3 tablespoons fresh chopped sweet basil

3 basil leaves for garnish (roll leaves and thinly slice)

**DIRECTIONS:**

Place beans and broth in a large saucepan. Cover, and bring to a boil, reduce heat to low and simmer until done. Drain and set aside. Melt butter in a skillet over medium heat and add sugar, garlic, salt, pepper. Add tomatoes and basil, cook until soft, but still whole, then pour tomato mixture over the green beans, and toss. Garnish with basil slices.

# Sautéed Asparagus with Balsamic Vinegar

**INGREDIENTS:**

2 lbs. of asparagus – wood ends removed

1 teaspoon of Extra Virgin Olive Oil

1 tablespoon of unsalted butter

2 cloves finely chopped garlic

1 cup of Balsamic Vinegar

2 teaspoons of freshly chopped tarragon

2 teaspoons of freshly chopped parsley

**DIRECTIONS:**

In a large sauce pan on medium heat ad olive oil and butter, when butter has melted add garlic, asparagus, and balsamic. Cook on medium high flame, constantly mix the asparagus in the balsamic until the balsamic becomes thick and the asparagus becomes tender, but not too soft. Remove from heat add the herb, cover the pan and let sit for about 10 minutes giving the asparagus time to absorb the flavors.

NOTE: This can also be cooked in the oven on a baking sheet at 375° for 20 minutes or until vegetables are tender.

# Succotash

It was my 6th season of gardening when I decided to plant some corn and I have not planted a garden without corn on the cob since. There is nothing like, planting those seeds and watching those little sprout grow into tall stalks of beautiful Silver Queen corn.

Then the reward of harvesting and shucking; then I blanch the ears of corn, remove the kernels from the cob and package it in Ziploc baggies – 2 cups per bag and we have "fresh-frozen" corn for the whole fall and winter seasons and … some great succotash.

## INGREDIENTS:

1-1lb bag frozen butter beans

2 cups of corn

½ stick of unsalted butter

4 tablespoons fresh parsley – finely chopped

1 teaspoon kosher salt

2 teaspoons coarse black pepper

## DIRECTIONS:

In medium sauce pan add beans and corn add just enough to cover the vegetables. Bring to boil, reduce heat add salt, pepper and butter, simmer for about 20 minutes, until beans are tender, then add parsley and serve.

This has been a great journey, sharing some of my favorite recipes and the juices
are still flowing. While writing this recipe book, I continued to cook!

Look for my next books with Quiche and Salad, Soup, Stew and Chili, Sandwiches and Burgers,

Cooking International and Seafood Delights and Appetizers.

Thank you all very much!

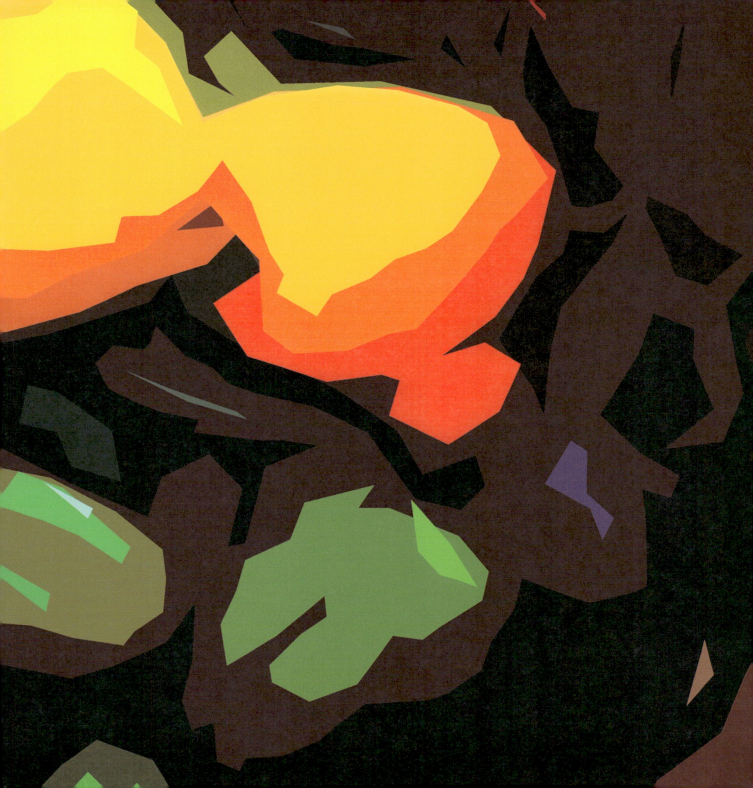

Printed in the United States
By Bookmasters